The Complete Dash Diet Meat & Seafood Cookbook

Amazing Dash Diet Meat & Seafood Recipes For Weight Loss

Peter Haley

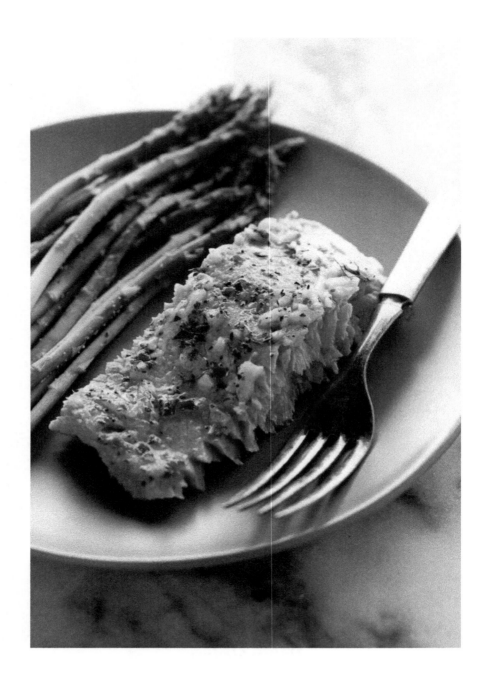

Table of contents

Friendly Chipotle Copycat

Prep Time: 5 mins

Servings: 6

Cooking: 55 mins

Ingredients:

- 3 lb of grass-fed chuck roast large chunks
- 1 large sized onion peeled and sliced up
- 6 garlic cloves
- 2 cans of 4 ounce of green chilies
- 1 tbsp of oregano
- 1 tsp of flavored vinegar
- 1 tsp of pepper
- 3 dried chipotle peppers with the stems removed broken up into small pieces
- Juice of 3 limes
- 3 tbsp of coconut vinegar
- 1 tbsp of cumin
- ½ a cup of water

Directions:

1. Add the listed Ingredients to your Instant Pot
2. Stir and lock up the lid , cook on HIGH pressure for 50 mins
3. Release the pressure naturally over 10 mins
4. Remove the lid and shred using a fork
5. Set your pot to Saute mode and reduce for 30 mins

Nutrition:

- Calories: 452
- Fat: 22g
- Carbs: 12g
- Protein: 52g

Ground Beef with Beans and Tomatoes

Prep Time: 15 mins

Servings: 6

Cooking: 30 mins

Ingredients:

- 1 tsp of olive oil
- 1 lb of lean ground beef
- 1 chopped medium onion
- 1 tbsp of minced garlic
- 1 tsp of dried thyme
- 1 tsp of dried oregano
- ½ a lb of green beans, ends trimmed and cut up into 1 inch pieces
- 2 can of petite diced tomatoes with juice
- 2 cans of beef broth
- Flavored vinegar and pepper as needed

Directions:

1. Set your pot to Saute mode and add oil, allow the oil to heat up. Add ground beef and stir well as it cooks
2. Once the beef is browned up, add chopped onion, dried thyme, minced garlic, dried oregano and cook for 3 mins
3. Add petite-dice tomatoes alongside the juice and beef broth
4. Allow them to heat for a while
5. Trim the beans on both ends and cut into 1 inch pieces
6. Add beans to your pot
7. Lock up the lid and cook on SOUP mode for 30 mins
8. Perform a quick release
9. Season with flavored vinegar and pepper
10. Serve freshly with a grating of parmesan

Nutrition:

- Calories: 327
- Fat: 24g
- Carbs: 12g
- Protein: 19g

Lamb Spare Ribs

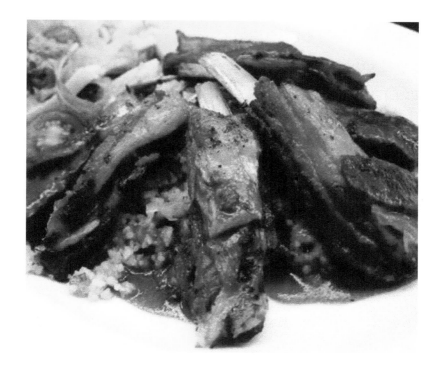

Prep Time: 5 mins

Servings: 5

Cooking: 20 mins

Ingredients:

- 2.5 lbs of pastured lamb spare ribs
- 2 tsps of kosher flavored vinegar
- 1 tbsp of curry powder

For the sauce

- 1 t tbsp of coconut oil
- 1 large sized coarsely chopped onion
- ½ a lb of minced garlic
- 1 tbsp of curry powder
- 1 tbsp of kosher flavored vinegar
- Juice from about 1 lemon
- 1 and a 1/4th cup of divided cilantro
- 4 thinly sliced scallion

Directions:

1. Take a bowl and add spare ribs
2. Season with 2 tsp of vinegar, 1 tsp of curry powder and mix well
3. Cover it up and let them freeze for at least 1 hour
4. Set your pot to Saute mode and add coconut oil
5. Add spare ribs and allow them to brown
6. Once done, transfer them to another plate
7. Take a blender and add tomatoes and onion and blend them well to a paste

8. Add the minced garlic to your instant pot (still in Saute mode)

9. Keep stirring the garlic while carefully poring the prepared paste

10. Add curry powder, chopped up cilantro , flavored vinegar and lemon juice .Allow the whole mixture to come to a boil

11. Add spare ribs and stir until it is coated well

12. Lock up the lid and cook for 20 mins at HIGH pressure

13. Allow the pressure to release naturally once done

14. Scoop out the grease and season with some flavored vinegar

Nutrition:

- Calories: 165
- Fats: 14g
- Carbs:5g
- Fiber:2g

Curry Lamb shanks

Prep Time: 35 mins

Servings: 5

Cooking: 45 mins

Ingredients:

- 3 lb of lamb shanks
- Amount of Kosher Flavored vinegar
- Freshly ground portions of black pepper
- 2 tbsp of well divided ghee
- 2 roughly chopped up medium sized carrots
- 2 celery roughly chopped up celery stalks
- 1 roughly chopped up large sized onion
- 1 tbsp of tomato paste
- 3 cloves of peeled and smashed garlic
- 1 cup of bone broth
- 1 tsp of Red Boast Fish Sauce
- 1 tbsp of vinegar

Directions:

1. Season the shanks with pepper and flavored vinegar
2. Set your pot to Saute mode and add ghee, allow the ghee to melt and heat up
3. Add shanks and cook for 8-10 mins until a nice brown texture appears
4. In the meantime, chop the vegetables
5. Once you have a nice brown texture on your lamb, remove it from the Instant Pot and keep it on the side
6. Add vegetables and season with flavored vinegar and pepper
7. Add a tbsp of ghee and mix
8. Add vegetables, garlic clove, tomato paste and give it a nice stir
9. Add shanks and pour broth, vinegar, fish sauce
10. Sprinkle a bit of pepper and lock up the lid
11. Cook on HIGH pressure for 45 mins
12. Release the pressure naturally over 10 mins

Nutrition:

- Calories: 377
- Fats: 16g
- Carbs: 10g
- Fiber: 2g

Moroccan Lamb Tajine

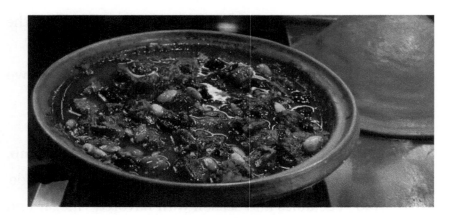

Prep Time: 10 mins

Cooking time: 50 mins

Servings: 4

Ingredients:

- 2 and a /13 lb of lamb shoulder
- 1 tsp of cinnamon powder
- 1 tsp of ginger powder
- 1 tsp of turmeric powder
- 2 cloves of crushed garlic

- 3 tbsp of olive oil
- 10 ounce of prunes pitted and soaked
- 1 cup of vegetable stock
- 2 medium roughly sliced onion
- 1 piece of bay leaf
- 1 stick of cinnamon
- 1 tsp of pepper
- 1 and a ½ tsp of flavored vinegar
- 3 and a ½ ounce of almonds
- 1 tbsp of sesame seeds

Directions:

1. Take a bowl and add ground cinnamon, ginger, turmeric, garlic and 2 spoons of olive oil
2. Make a paste
3. Cover the lamb with the paste
4. Take a bowl and add dried prunes with boiling water and cover, keep it on the side
5. Set your pot to Saute mode and add olive oil
6. Add onion and cook for 3 mins
7. Transfer the onion to a bowl and keep it on the side
8. Add meat and brown all sides for about 10 mins
9. Deglaze using vegetable stock
10. Add onions, cinnamon stick, bay leaf

11. Lock up the lid and cook on HIGH pressure for 35 mins
12. Release the pressure naturally
13. Add rinsed and drained prunes and set the pot to Saute mode
14. Reduce the liquid by simmer for 5 mins
15. Discard the bay leaf and sprinkle toasted almonds alongside sesame seeded

Nutrition:

- Protein: 6.2g
- Carbs: 2.0g
- Fats: 11.8g
- Calories: 134

Quick Jalapeno Crisps

Prep Time: 35 mins

Servings: 20

Cooking: 25 mins

Ingredients:

- 5 sliced jalapenos
- Tabasco sauce for serving
- ½ tsp onion powder
- 8 oz grated parmesan cheese
- 3 tbsp olive oil

Directions:
1. Mix the jalapeno slices with salt, pepper, oil and onion powder, toss to coat and arrange on a lined baking sheet
2. Preheat your oven to a temperature of 450F and introduce the mix and bake for 15 mins

3. Take jalapeno slices out of the oven, set them aside and allow them to cool down
4. In another bowl, mix pepper slices with the cheese and compress well
5. Place all the slices on another lined baking sheet and introduce into the oven again and bake for 10 mins more
6. Leave jalapenos to cool down
7. Arrange on a plate and serve with Tabasco sauce on the side

Nutrition:

- Calories 50
- Fat 1g
- Carbs 3g
- Protein 2g

Crispy Egg Chips

Prep Time: 15 mins

Servings: 2

Cooking: 15 mins

Ingredients:

- 4 eggs whites
- 2 tbsp shredded parmesan
- ½ tbsp water

Directions:

1. Put the egg whites with water in a bowl and mix and whisk well
2. Spoon this into a muffin pan, sprinkle cheese on top
3. introduce the mix in the oven at 400 degrees F and bake for 15 mins
4. Move the egg white chips to a platter and serve with a dip on the side

Nutrition:

- Calories 120
- Fiber 1
- Fat 2
- Carbs 2g
- Protein 7g

Marinated beef Kebabs

Prep Time: 30 mins

Servings: 6

Cooking: 10 mins

Ingredients:

- 1 red/green/orange bell pepper, cut into chunks
- 2 lbs sirloin steak, cut into medium cubes
- 4 minced garlic cloves
- ¼ cup tamari sauce
- ½ cup olive oil
- 1/4 cup lemon juice
- 1 red onion, cut into chunks
- 2½ tbsp Worcestershire sauce
- 2 tbsp Dijon mustard

Directions:

1. Mix the Worcestershire sauce with garlic, mustard, tamari, lemon juice and oil and stir until even

2. Include beef, bell peppers and onion chunks to this mix, toss to coat and set aside for a few mins
3. Arrange bell pepper, meat cubes and onion chunks on skewers alternating colors
4. Place the mix on your preheated grill of over medium-high heat and cook for 5 mins on each side.
5. Move to a platter and serve as a summer appetizer.

Nutrition:

- Calories 246
- Fiber 1g
- Carbs 4g
- Fat 12g
- Protein 26g

Cowboy Caviar Salad

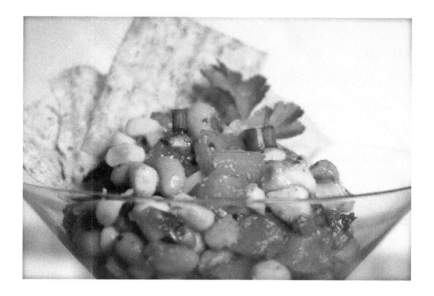

Prep Time: 6 mins

Servings: 16

Ingredients:

- mayonnaise-¾ cup
- 8 eggs, hardboiled, peeled and mashed with a fork
- 1 yellow onion, finely chopped
- 4 oz red caviar

- toast baguette slices for serving
- 4 oz black caviar

Directions:

1. Mix in a bowl mashed eggs with mayonnaise, salt, pepper and onion and stir well
2. Spread eggs salad on toasted baguette slices
3. Add caviar at the top of the slices.

Nutrition:

- Calories 122
- Fiber 1g
- Carbs 4g
- Protein 7g
- Fat 8g

Asparagus And Lemon Salmon Dish

Prep Time: 5 mins

Servings: 3

Cooking: 15 mins

Ingredients:

- 2 salmon fillets, 6 oz each, skin on
- Sunflower seeds to taste
- 1 lb asparagus, trimmed
- 2 cloves garlic, minced
- 3 tbsps almond butter
- ¼ cup cashew cheese

Directions:

1. Pre-heat your oven to 400F
2. Line a baking sheet with oil
3. Take a kitchen towel and pat your salmon dry, season as needed

4. Put salmon around baking sheet and arrange asparagus around it
5. Place a pan over medium heat and melt almond butter
6. Add garlic and cook for 3 mins until garlic browns slightly
7. Drizzle sauce over salmon
8. Sprinkle salmon with cheese and bake for 12 mins until salmon looks cooked all the way and is flaky

Nutrition:

- Calories 131
- Fiber 1g
- Carbs 7g
- Protein 8g
- Fat 8g

Spicy Baked Shrimp

Prep Time: 10 mins

Servings: 4

Cooking: 25 mins + 2-4 hours

Ingredients:

- ½ oz large shrimp, peeled and deveined
- Cooking spray as needed
- 1 tsp low sodium coconut aminos
- 1 tsp parsley
- ½ tsp olive oil
- ½ tbsp honey
- 1 tbsp lemon juice

Directions:

1. Pre-heat your oven to 450 degrees F
2. Take a baking dish and grease it well
3. Mix in all the ingredients: and toss

4. Transfer to oven and bake for 8 mins until shrimp turn pink

Nutrition:

- Calories 135
- Fiber 1g
- Carbs 8g
- Protein 10g
- Fat 8g

Shallot and Tuna

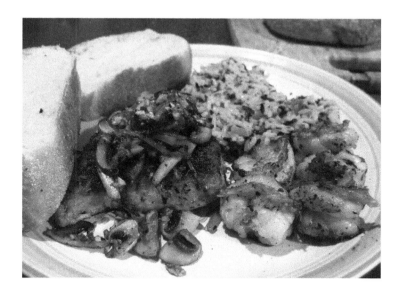

Prep Time: 10 mins

Servings: 4

Cooking: 15 mins

Ingredients:

- 4 tuna fillets, boneless and skinless
- 1 tbsp olive oil

- 2 shallots, chopped
- 2 tbsps lime juice
- Pinch of pepper
- 1 tsp sweet paprika
- ½ cup low sodium chicken stock

Directions:

1. Take a pan and place it over medium heat, add shallots and Sauté for 3 mins
2. Add fish, cook for 4 mins
3. Add remaining Ingredients; cook for 3 mins

Nutrition:

- Calories 121
- Fiber 1g
- Carbs 8g
- Protein 7g
- Fat 8g

Brazilian Shrimp Stew

Prep Time: 20 mins

Servings: 4

Cooking: 25 mins

Ingredients:

- 4 tbsps lime juice
- 1 and ½ tbsp cumin, ground
- 1 and ½ tbsp paprika
- 2 and ½ tsps garlic, minced
- 1 and ½ tsp pepper
- 2 lbs tilapia fillets, cut into bits
- 1 large onion, chopped
- 3 large bell pepper, cut into strips
- 1 can (14 oz) tomato, drained
- 1 can (14 oz) coconut milk
- Handful of cilantro, chopped

Directions:

1. Take a large sized bowl and add lime juice, cumin, paprika, garlic, pepper and mix well
2. Add tilapia and coat it up
3. Cover and allow it to marinate for 20 mins
4. Set your pot to HIGH and add olive oil
5. Add onions and cook for 3 mins until tender
6. Add pepper strips, tilapia, and tomatoes to a skillet
7. Pour coconut milk and cover, simmer for 20 mins
8. Add cilantro during the final few mins

Nutrition:

- Calories 121
- Fiber 1g
- Carbs 8g
- Protein 7g
- Fat 8g

Heart-Warming Medi Tilapia

Prep Time: 15 mins

Servings: 4

Cooking: 15 mins

Ingredients:

- 3 tbsps sun-dried tomatoes, packed in oil, drained and chopped
- 1 tbsp capers, drained
- 2 tilapia fillets
- 1 tbsp oil from sun-dried tomatoes
- 2 tbsps kalamata olives, chopped and pitted

Directions:

1. Pre-heat your oven to 372 degrees F
2. Take a small sized bowl and add sun-dried tomatoes, olives, capers and stir well
3. Keep the mixture on the side

4. Take a baking sheet and transfer the tilapia fillets and arrange them side by side
5. Drizzle olive oil all over them
6. Bake in your oven for 10-15 mins
7. After 10 mins, check the fish for a "Flaky" texture
8. Once cooked properly, top the fish with tomato mixture and serve!

Nutrition:

- Calories 131
- Fiber 1g
- Carbs 7g
- Protein 8g
- Fat 8g

Lemon Cod

Prep Time: 15 mins

Servings: 2

Cooking: 20 mins

Ingredients:

- 4 tbsps almond butter, divided
- 4 thyme sprigs, fresh and divided
- 4 tsps lemon juice, fresh and divided
- 4 cod fillets, 6 oz each
- Sunflower seeds to taste

Directions:

1. Pre-heat your oven to 400 degrees F.
2. Season cod fillets with sunflower seeds on both side.
3. Take four pieces of foil, each foil should be 3 times bigger than fillets.
4. Divide fillets between the foils and top with almond butter, lemon juice, thyme.

5. Fold to form a pouch and transfer pouches to the baking sheet.
6. Bake for 20 mins.
7. Open and let the steam get out.

Nutrition:

- Calories 122
- Fiber 1g
- Carbs 4g
- Protein 7g
- Fat 8g

Lemon And Garlic Scallops

Prep Time: 10 mins

Servings: 4

Cooking: 5 mins

Ingredients:

1. 1 tbsp olive oil
2. 1 and ¼ lbs dried scallops
3. 2 tbsps all-purpose flour
4. ¼ tsp sunflower seeds
5. 4-5 garlic cloves, minced
6. 1 scallion, chopped
7. 1 pinch of ground sage
8. 1 lemon juice
9. 2 tbsps parsley, chopped

Directions:

1. Take a non-stick skillet and place it over medium-high heat

2. Add oil and allow the oil to heat up
3. Take a medium sized bowl and add scallops alongside sunflower seeds and flour
4. Place the scallops in the skillet and add scallions, garlic, and sage
5. Saute for 3-4 mins until they show an opaque texture
6. Stir in lemon juice and parsley
7. Remove heat and serve hot!

Nutrition:

- Calories 121
- Fiber 1g
- Carbs 8g
- Protein 7g
- Fat 8g

Cajun Snow Crab

Prep Time: 10 mins

Servings: 4

Cooking: 10 mins

Ingredients:

- 1 lemon, fresh and quartered
- 3 tbsps Cajun seasoning
- 2 bay leaves
- 4 snow crab legs, precooked and defrosted
- Golden ghee

Directions:

1. Take a large pot and fill it about halfway with sunflower seeds and water
2. Bring the water to a boil
3. Squeeze lemon juice into pot and toss in remaining lemon quarters
4. Add bay leaves and Cajun seasoning

5. Season for 1 minute
6. Add crab legs and boil for 8 mins (make sure to keep them submerged the whole time)
7. Melt ghee in microwave and use as dipping sauce, enjoy!

Nutrition:

- Calories 142
- Fiber 4g
- Carbs 10g
- Protein 9g
- Fat 8g

Calamari Citrus

Prep Time: 10 mins

Servings: 4

Cooking: 5 mins

Ingredients:

- 1 lime, sliced
- 1 lemon, sliced
- 2 lbs calamari tubes and tentacles, sliced
- Pepper to taste
- ¼ cup olive oil
- 2 garlic cloves, minced
- 3 tbsps lemon juice
- 1 orange, peeled and cut into segments
- 2 tbsps cilantro, chopped

Directions:

1. Take a bowl and add calamari, pepper, lime slices, lemon slices, orange slices, garlic, oil, cilantro, lemon juice and toss well
2. Take a pan and place it over medium-high heat
3. Add calamari mix and cook for 5 mins
4. Divide into bowls and serve

Nutrition:

- Calories 121
- Fiber 1g
- Carbs 8g
- Protein 7g
- Fat 8g

Lasagna

Prep Time: 15 mins

Servings: 8

Cooking: 25 mins

Ingredients:

- 3 cup shredded mozzare lla cheese
- 1 cup cottage cheese
- ¾ lb. lasagna noodles
- 3 ½ cup Water
- 8 oz unsalted tomato sauce
- 6 oz unsalted tomato paste
- ¾ tsp garlic powder
- ¾ tsp Oregano
- 1½ tsp dried basil
- 1 sliced onion
- 1 lb. extra-lean ground beef

Directions:

1. Lightly coat a 10-14 cooking pan with cooking spray. Also, preheat the oven to 325 F

2. Now, for the sauce, put a large saucepan on the stove and place the ground beef and onion in it and cook until the meet is golden brown

3. Once brown, drain the pan and then add the water, tomato sauce, tomato paste, garlic powder, oregano, and basil and stir until it comes to a boil. Reduce the heat and simmer for 10 mins

4. In the cooking pan, place a half cup of the mixture on the bottom of the pan.

5. On top of the mixture, place a layer of the uncooked lasagna noodles and then add another layer of the mixture, as well as a cup of mozzarella cheese and a third of a cup of cottage cheese.

6. Do the same for the remaining mixture.

7. Place aluminum foil on top of the lasagna and put it into the oven.

8. Bake the lasagna for an hour and fifteen mins or until the cheese is brown

9. Let the lasagna cool before serving.

Nutrition:

- Calories 425
- Carbs 42g
- Fat 13g
- Protein 33g

Shrimp And Avocado Dish

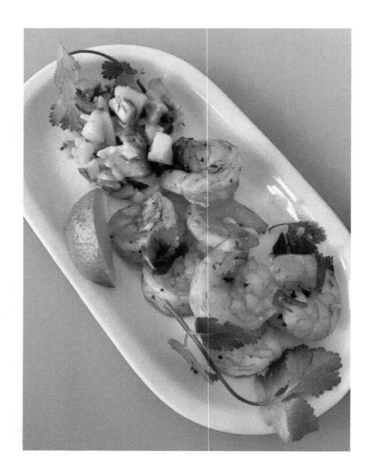

Prep Time: 10 mins

Servings: 8

Ingredients:

- 2 green onions, chopped
- 2 avocados, pitted, peeled and cut into chunks
- 2 tbsps cilantro, chopped
- 1 cup shrimp, cooked, peeled and deveined
- Pinch of pepper

Directions:

1. Take a bowl and add cooked shrimp, avocado, green onions, cilantro, pepper
2. Toss well and serve

Nutrition:

- Calories 121
- Fiber 1g
- Carbs 8g
- Protein 7g
- Fat 8g

Fresh Calamari

Prep Time: 10 mins +1 hour marinating

Servings: 4 | **Cooking:** 8 mins

Ingredients:

- 2 tbsp extra virgin olive oil
- 1 tsp chili powder
- ½ tsp ground cumin
- Zest of 1 lime
- Juice of 1 lime
- Dash of sea sunflower seeds
- 1 and ½ lbs squid, cleaned and split open, with tentacles cut into ½ inch rounds
- 2 tbsps cilantro, chopped
- 2 tbsps red bell pepper, minced

Directions:

1. Take a medium bowl and stir in olive oil, chili powder, cumin, lime zest, sea sunflower seeds, lime juice and pepper

2. Add squid and let it marinade and stir to coat, coat and let it refrigerate for 1 hour
3. Pre-heat your oven to broil
4. Arrange squid on a baking sheet, broil for 8 mins turn once until tender
5. Garnish the broiled calamari with cilantro and red bell pepper

Nutrition:

- Calories 121
- Fiber 1g
- Carbs 8g
- Protein 7g
- Fat 8g

Deep Fried Prawn And Rice Croquettes

Prep Time: 25 mins

Servings: 4

Cooking: 13 mins

Ingredients:

- 2 tbsps almond butter
- ½ onion, chopped
- 4 oz shrimp, peeled and chopped
- 2 tbsps all-purpose flour
- 1 tbsp white wine
- ½ cup almond milk
- 2 tbsps almond milk
- 2 cups cooked rice
- 1 tbsp parmesan, grated
- 1 tsp fresh dill, chopped
- 1 tsp sunflower seeds
- Ground pepper as needed
- Vegetable oil for frying

- 3 tbsps all-purpose flour
- 1 whole egg
- ½ cup breadcrumbs

Directions:

1. Take a large skillet and place it over medium heat, add almond butter and let it melt

2. Add onion, cook and stir for 5 mins

3. Add shrimp and cook for 1-2 mins

4. Stir in 2 tbsps flour, white wine, pour in almond milk gradually and cook for 3-5 mins until the sauce thickens

5. Remove white sauce from heat and stir in rice, mix evenly

6. Add parmesan, cheese, dill, sunflower seeds, pepper and let it cool for 15 mins

7. Heat oil in large saucepan and bring it to 350 degrees F

8. Take a bowl and whisk in egg, spread bread crumbs on a plate

9. Form rice mixture into 8 balls and roll 1 ball in flour, dip in egg and coat with crumbs, repeat with all balls

10. Deep fry balls for 3 mins

Nutrition:

- Calories 180
- Fiber 1g
- Carbs 10g
- Protein 12g
- Fat 10g

Thai Pumpkin Seafood Stew

Prep Time: 5 mins

Servings: 4

Cooking: 35 mins

Ingredients:

- 1 and ½ tbsps fresh galangal, chopped
- 1 tsp lime zest
- 1 small kabocha squash
- 32 medium sized mussels, fresh
- 1 lb shrimp
- 16 thai leaves
- 1 can coconut milk
- 1 tbsp lemongrass, minced
- 4 garlic cloves, roughly chopped
- 32 medium clams, fresh
- 1 and ½ lbs fresh salmon
- 2 tbsp coconut oil
- Pepper to taste

Directions:

1. Add coconut milk, lemongrass, galangal, garlic, lime leaves in a small-sized saucepan, bring to a boil.
2. Let it simmer for 25 mins.
3. Strain mixture through fine sieve into the large soup pot and bring to a simmer.
4. Add oil to a pan and heat up, add Kabocha squash.
5. Saute for 5 mins.
6. Add mix to coconut mix.
7. Heat oil in a pan and add fish shrimp, season with salt and pepper, cook for 4 mins.
8. Add mixture to coconut milk mix alongside clams and mussels.
9. Simmer for 8 mins, garnish with basil and enjoy!

Nutrition:

- Calories 121
- Fiber 1g
- Carbs 8g
- Protein 7g
- Fat 8g

Blackened Tilapia

Prep Time: 9 mins

Servings: 2

Cooking: 9 mins

Ingredients:

- 1 cup of cauliflower, chopped
- 1 tsp of red pepper flakes
- 1 tbsp of Italian seasoning
- 1 tbsp of garlic, minced
- 6 ounce of tilapia
- 1 cup of English cucumber, chopped with peel
- 2 tbsp of olive oil
- 1 sprig dill, chopped
- 1 tsp of stevia
- 3 tbsp of lime juice
- 2 tbsp of Cajun blackened seasoning

Directions:

1. Take a bowl and add the seasoning **Ingredients:** (except Cajun).
2. Add a tbsp of oil and whip.
3. Pour dressing over cauliflower and cucumber.
4. Brush the fish with olive oil on both sides.
5. Take a skillet and grease it well with 1 tbsp of olive oil.
6. Press Cajun seasoning on both sides of fish.
7. Cook fish for 3 mins per side

Nutrition:

- Calories 121
- Fiber 1g
- Carbs 8g
- Protein 7g
- Fat 8g

Steak Tacos

Prep Time: 15 mins

Servings: 4

Cooking: 13 mins

Ingredients:

- 1 lb beef flank (or round) steak
- 1 tsp chili powder
- 1 tsp olive oil
- 1 green bell pepper, cored and coarsely chopped
- 1 red onion, coarsely chopped
- 8 (6-inch) corn tortillas, warm
- 2 tbsp freshly squeezed lime juice
- Optional for servings: 1 avocado, sliced, and coarsely chopped cilantro

Directions:

1. Rub the steak with chili powder (and salt and pepper, if desired).

2. Heat olive oil in a large skillet over medium-high heat.
3. Add steak and cook for 6 to 8 mins on each side or until it is done. Remove from heat.
4. Place steak on a plate and cover with aluminum foil. Let rest for 5 mins.
5. Add the bell pepper and onion to skillet. Cook on medium heat, stirring frequently, for 3 to 5 mins or until onion is translucent. Remove from heat.
6. Cut steak against the grain into thin slices.
7. Top tortillas evenly with beef, onion mixture, and lime juice. Garnish with avocado and cilantro, if desired.

Nutrition:

- Calories 358
- Fat 12g
- Carbs 34g
- Fiber 2g
- Protein 28g

Beef-and-Bean Chili

Prep Time: 5 mins

Servings: 4

Cooking: 20 mins

Ingredients:

- 1 lb lean or extra-lean ground beef
- 1 yellow onion, diced
- 3 (15 oz) cans salt-free diced tomatoes with green chilies
- 2 (15 oz) cans beans, drained and rinsed (whatever you desire: black, red, pinto, kidney, etc)
- 2 tbsp chili powder
- Optional: 1 (10-ounce) package frozen spinach

Directions:

1. In a large stockpot, cook the beef over medium-high heat until browned, stirring frequently

2. Using a slotted spoon, transfer the cooked beef to a separate plate and set aside

3. Reserve 1 tbsp of grease in the stockpot and discard the rest.

4. Add the onion to the stockpot and sauté for 4 to 5 mins until soft.

5. Add the tomatoes with green chilies, beans, chili powder, and cooked beef to the stockpot. Stir to combine. Bring to a boil and then reduce heat to medium-low. Cover and simmer for 10 mins.

Nutrition:

- Calories 429
- Fat 10g
- Carbs 47g
- Fiber 16g
- Protein 38g

Asian Pork Tenderloin

Prep Time: 10 mins

Servings: 4

Cooking: 15 mins

Ingredients:

- 2 tbsp sesame seeds
- 1 tsp ground coriander
- 1/8 tsp cayenne pep per
- 1/8 tsp celery seed
- 1/2 tsp minced onion
- 1/4 tsp ground cumin
- 1/8 tsp ground cinnamon
- 1 tbsp sesame oil
- 1-lb pork tenderloin, sliced into 4 4-ounce portions

Directions:

1. Set the oven to heat at 400°F. Grease a baking dish with cooking oil.

2. Toast the sesame seeds in a dry frying pan until golden brown.
3. Transfer the sesame seeds to a bowl and set it aside.
4. Combine coriander with celery seed, cinnamon, toasted sesame seeds, cumin, sesame oil, and minced onion in a bowl.
5. Place the pork tenderloin in a baking dish and rub them with pepper mixture.
6. Bake them for 15 mins.

Nutrition:

- Calories 248
- Fat 13.8 g
- Carbs 1.1 g
- Fiber 3.1g
- Protein 55.9 g

Curried Pork Tenderloin in Apple Cider

Prep Time: 6 mins

Servings: 6

Cooking: 30 mins

Ingredients:

- 16 oz pork tenderloin, cut into 6 pieces
- 1 1/2 tbsp curry powder
- 1 tbsp extra-virgin olive oil
- 2 medium yellow onions, chopped (about 2 cups)
- 2 cups apple cider, divided
- 1 tart apple, peeled, seeded, and chopped into chunks
- 1 tbsp cornstarch

Directions:

1. Rub the pork tenderloin with curry powder and let it rest for 15 mins.
2. Preheat a skillet with olive oil on medium heat.

3. Sear the tenderloin for 10 mins per side and then transfer it to a plate.
4. Add onions to the same skillet and sauté until golden and soft.
5. Stir in 1 ½ cups apple cider and cook until it is reduced to half.
6. Add chopped apples, remaining apple cider, and cornstarch.
7. Stir and then cook the mixture for 2 mins until it thickens.
8. Return the tenderloin to the sauce.
9. Let it cook for 5 mins in the sauce.

Nutrition:

- Calories 244
- Fat 14.8 g
- Carbs 19.4 g
- Fiber 1.3 g
- Protein 10.2 g

New York Strip Steak

Prep Time: 15 mins

Servings: 2

Cooking: 20 mins

Ingredients:

- 2 New York strip steaks, 4 oz each, trimmed of all visible fat
- 1 tsp trans-free margarine
- 3 garlic cloves, chopped
- 2 oz sliced shiitake mushrooms
- 2 oz button mushrooms
- 1/4 tsp thyme
- 1/4 tsp rosemary
- 1/4 cup whiskey

Directions:

1. Preheat a charcoal grill or broiler. Grease the racks with cooking spray.

2. Place the greased rack about 4 inches away from the heat source.
3. Grill the steaks in the preheated grill for 10 mins per side.
4. Sauté garlic with mushrooms, rosemary, and thyme in a greased skillet.
5. Cook for 2 mins and then stir in whiskey after removing the pan from the heat.
6. Pour this sauce over steaks.

Nutrition:

- Calories 330
- Fat 9.8 g
- Carbs 21.1 g
- Fiber 3.1 g
- Protein 44 g

Mediterranean Pork Pasta

Prep Time: 15 mins

Servings: 4

Cooking: 15 mins

Ingredients:

- 2 cups dry whole-wheat penne pasta (8 oz)
- 1 tbsp olive oil
- 1 tsp garlic, minced (about 1/2 clove)
- 8 oz white button mushrooms, rinsed and cut into quarters
- 1/2 bag (8 oz bag) sundried tomato halves, cut into thin strips
- 1/2 jar (8 oz jar) artichoke hearts in water, drained, cut into quarters
- 2 cups low-sodium beef broth
- 2 tbsps cornstarch
- 12 oz stir-fry pork strips, sliced into 12 strips (or, slice 3 4-oz boneless pork chops into thin strips)

- 1/4 cup fat-free evaporated milk
- 2 tbsps fresh parsley, rinsed, dried, and chopped (or 2 tsps dried)

Directions:

1. In a 4-quart saucepan, bring 3 quarts of water to a boil over high heat.
2. Add pasta, and cook according to package directions. Drain. (Set plain pasta aside for picky eaters—see Healthy Eating Two Ways suggestion below.)
3. Meanwhile, heat olive oil and garlic in a large sauté pan over medium heat. Cook until soft, but not browned (about 30 seconds).
4. Add mushrooms, and cook over medium heat until the mushrooms are soft and lightly browned.
5. Add sundried tomatoes and artichoke hearts. Toss gently to heat.
6. In a separate bowl, combine beef broth and cornstarch. Mix well.
7. Add broth mixture to the pan, and bring to a boil.
8. Add pork strips, evaporated milk, and parsley, and bring to a boil. Simmer gently for 3–5 mins (to a minimum internal temperature of 160 °F).
9. Add pasta, and toss well to mix.
10. Serve 2 cups of pasta and sauce per portion.

Nutrition:

- Calories 486
- Fat 11 g
- Protein 33 g
- Carbs 56 g

Pork Medallions with Herbs de Provence

Prep Time: 10 mins

Servings: 4

Cooking: 20 mins

Ingredients:

- 8 oz pork tenderloin, trimmed of visible fat and cut crosswise into 6 pieces
- 1/2 tsp herbs de Provence
- 1/4 cup dry white wine

Directions:

1. Season the pork with black pepper and place the meat between sheets of parchment paper.
2. Punch the pork pieces with a mallet into ¼ inch thickness.
3. Sear the seasoned pork in a greased skillet for 3 mins per side.

4. Remove it from the pan and drizzle with herbs de Provence.
5. Transfer the pork to the serving plate.
6. Add wine to the same skillet and scrape off the brown bits while stirring.
7. Pour this wine over the medallions.

Nutrition:

- Calories 120
- Fat 24 g
- Carbs 26.4 g
- Fiber 1.5 g
- Protein 23.4 g

Pork and Mint Corn

Prep Time: 10 mins

Servings: 4

Ingredients:

- 1 cup corn
- 1 tbsp chopped mint
- 1 cup low-sodium veggie stock
- Black pepper
- 1 tbsp olive oil
- 1 tsps. sweet paprika
- 4 pork chops

Directions:

1. Put the pork chops in a roasting pan, add the rest of the ingredients, toss, introduce in the oven and bake at 380 º F for 1 hour.
2. Divide everything between plates and serve.

Nutrition:

- Calories 356
- Fat 14 g
- Carbs 11.0 g
- Protein 1g

Pork Chops and Snow Peas

Prep Time: 10 mins

Servings: 4

Ingredients:

- 2 tbsp olive oil
- 1 cup low-sodium veggie stock
- 4 pork chops
- 1 cup snow peas
- 2 chopped shallots
- 1 tbsp chopped parsley
- 2 tbsp no-salt-added tomato paste

Directions:

1. Heat up a pan with the oil over medium heat, add the shallots, toss and sauté for 5 mins.
2. Add the pork chops and brown for 2 mins on each side.
3. Add the rest of the ingredients, bring to a simmer and cook over medium heat for 15 mins.
4. Divide the mix between plates and serve.

Nutrition:

- Calories 357
- Fat 27 g
- Carbs 7.7 g
- Protein 20.7 g

Pork Meatballs

Prep Time: 10 mins

Servings: 4

Ingredients:

- 2 tbsp avocado oil
- 1 tbsp chopped cilantro
- 3 tbsp almond flour
- 2 whisked egg
- 10 oz. no-salt-added canned tomato sauce
- Black pepper
- 2 lbs. ground pork

Directions:

1. In a bowl, combine the pork with the flour and the other ingredients: except the sauce and the oil, stir well and shape medium meatballs out of this mix.
2. Heat up a pan with the oil over medium heat, add the meatballs and brown for 3 mins on each side.
3. Add the sauce, toss gently, bring to a simmer and cook over medium heat for 20 mins more.

4. Divide everything into bowls and serve.

Nutrition:

- Calories 332
- Fat18 g
- Carbs 14.3 g
- Protein 25 g

Pork with Sprouts

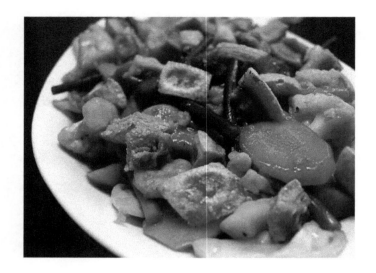

Prep Time: 10 mins

Servings: 4

Ingredients:

- 1 cup bean sprouts
- 1 cup low-sodium veggie stock
- 1 wedged yellow onion
- 2 tbsp olive oil
- 1 lb. pork chops

- Black pepper
- 2 tbsp drained capers

Directions:

1. Heat up a pan with the oil over medium-high heat, add the onion and the meat and brown for 5 mins.
2. Add the rest of the ingredients, introduce the pan in the oven and bake at 390 º F for 30 mins.
3. Divide everything between plates and serve.

Nutrition:

- Calories 324
- Fat 12.5 g
- Carbs 22.2 g
- Protein:15.6 g

Beef Stew with Fennel and Shallots

Prep Time: 10 mins

Servings: 6

Cooking: 1 hour

Ingredients:

- 1/3 cup chopped fresh parsley
- 3 Portobello mushrooms
- 18 small boiling onions
- 4 large red-skinned potatoes
- 4 large sliced carrots
- 3 cup vegetable stock
- 1 bay leaf
- 2 fresh thyme sprigs
- ¾ tsp ground black pepper
- 3 large shallots
- ½ fennel bulb
- 2 tbsp olive oil
- 1 lb. boneless lean beef stew meat

- 3 tbsp all-purpose flour

Directions:

1. Put the flour on a place and rolling the beef cubes in the flour
2. Using a large saucepan, pour the oil in and heat at medium heat
3. Once the beef is floured, put it into the sauce pan and cook until brown on all sides
4. Remove the beef and let cook elsewhere
5. Without changing the temperature, place the shallots and the fennel in the pan and cook until they are a light brown
6. Add the lay leaf, thyme sprigs, and a quarter of the pepper to the mix and let cook for a minute or two
7. Now, add the beef back into the pan with the vegetable stock and bring the mixture to a boil. After, reduce the heat and cover it while it simmers. Leave it like this for 30 mins
8. Once the meat is tender, add the mushrooms, onions, potatoes, and carrots
9. Stir the mixture and let simmer for another 30 mins
10. Pull the bay leaf and the thyme sprigs out of the stew and stir in the parsley and remaining pepper

Nutrition:

- Calories 244
- Fat 8g
- Carbs 22g
- Protein 21g

Grilled Portobello Mushroom Burger

Prep Time: 15 mins

Servings: 4

Cooking: 15 mins

Ingredients:

- 2 romaine lettuce leaves
- 4 slices of red onion
- 1 slices of tomato
- 4 whole-wheat toasted buns
- 2 tbsp olive oil
- ¼ tsp cayenne pepper
- 1 minced garlic clove
- 1 tbsp Sugar
- ½ cup water
- 1/3 cup balsamic vinegar
- 4 large Portobello mushroom caps

Directions:

1. The Portobello mushrooms need to be cleaned and their stems need to be removed and the caps need to be set aside

2. Now, in a small bowl the olive oil, cayenne pepper, garlic, sugar, water, and vinegar need to be mixed together and pored over top the mushroom caps

3. The caps need to be placed into a plastic container, covered, and placed into the refrigerator to marinate for an hour

4. Turn on the grill and lightly coat it in cooking spray— or, turn on the stove and coat a frying pan in the same substance

5. Fry or grill the mushrooms on medium heat, making sure to flip them often. Usually, it will take five mins on each side

6. Place the mushrooms on their own bun and top with half a lettuce leaf, one onion slice and one tomato slice.

Nutrition:

- Calories 301
- Fat 9g
- Carbs 45g
- Protein 10g

Pork and Green Onions

Prep Time: 10 mins

Servings: 5

Cooking: 10 mins

Ingredients:

- 1 tbsp avocado oil
- 4 minced garlic cloves
- 1 lb. cubed pork meat
- 1 chopped green onion bunch
- Black pepper
- 1 cup low-sodium tomato sauce
- 1 chopped yellow onion

Directions:

1. Heat up a pan with the oil over medium-high heat, add the onion and green onions, stir and cook for 5 mins.
2. Add the meat, stir and cook for 5 mins more.

3. Add the rest of the ingredients, toss and cook over medium heat for 30 mins more.
4. Divide everything into bowls and serve.

Nutrition:

- Calories 206
- Fat 8.6 g
- Carbs 7.2 g
- Protein 23.4 g

Chili Verde

Prep Time: 10 mins

Servings: 4

Cooking: 55 mins

Ingredients:

- 1 lb fresh tomatillos, husks removed, washed, and cut into quarters
- 3 Anaheim chilies, roasted, peeled, seeded, and diced
- 3 green onions, sliced
- 2 cloves garlic, chopped
- 1 jalapeño pepper, seeded and diced
- 2 tbsps fresh lime juice
- 1 tsp sugar
- 2 tsps oil
- 1-1/2 lbs lean pork tenderloin, cut into 3/4-inch chunks
- 1/4 cup chopped fresh cilantro

Directions:

1. Place tomatillos in a medium saucepan with a small amount of water. Cover and simmer for about 5 mins until soft.

2. Drain tomatillos and place in a blender container with the Anaheim chilies, green onions, garlic, and jalapeño pepper. Blend on low speed until fairly smooth. Stir in lime juice and sugar and pour back into saucepan; set aside.

3. Heat oil in a large skillet. Add pork to skillet; cook and stir over high heat for about 5 mins to brown; add to the pan with the sauce. Bring to a boil; reduce heat and simmer, covered, for 40 mins.

4. Remove cover and cook for 10 mins more. Stir in cilantro and salt. Serve with 1/2 cup cooked brown rice.

Nutrition:

- Calories 413
- Carbs 35 g
- Fiber 6 g
- Protein 43 g
- Fat 11 g

Pork and Carrots Soup

Prep Time: 10 mins

Servings: 4

Ingredients:

- 1 lb. cubed pork stew meat
- 1 tbsp chopped cilantro
- 1 tbsp olive oil
- 1 chopped red onion
- 1 cup tomato puree
- 1 quart low-sodium beef stock
- 1 lb. sliced carrots

Directions:

1. Heat up a pot with the oil over medium-high heat, add the onion and the meat and brown for 5 mins.
2. Add the rest of the ingredients: except the cilantro, bring to a simmer, reduce heat to medium, and boil the soup for 20 mins.

3. Ladle into bowls and serve for lunch with the cilantro sprinkled on top.

Nutrition:

- Calories 354
- Fat 14.6 g
- Carbs 19.3 g
- Protein 36 g

Chili Pork

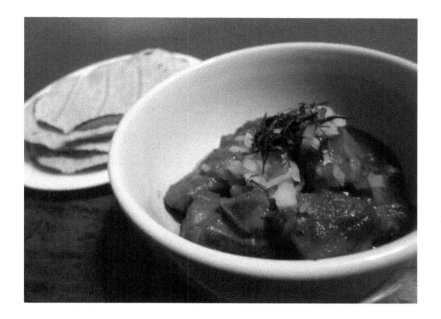

Prep Time: 10 mins

Servings: 4

Ingredients:

- 1 tbsp chopped oregano
- 2 lbs. cubed pork stew meat
- 1 chopped yellow onion
- 2 tbsp chili paste

- 2 minced garlic cloves
- 2 cup low-sodium beef stock
- 1 tbsp olive oil

Directions:

1. Heat up a pot with the oil, over medium-high heat, add the onion and the garlic, stir and sauté for 5 mins.
2. Add the meat and brown it for 5 mins more.
3. Add the rest of the ingredients, bring to a simmer and cook over medium heat for 20 mins more.
4. Divide the mix into bowls and serve.

Nutrition:

- Calories 363
- Fat 8.6 g
- Carbs 17.3 g
- Protein 18.4 g

Asian Pork Tenderloin

Prep Time: 20 mins

Servings: 4

Cooking: 15 mins

Ingredients:

- 1 lb. pork tenderloin
- 1 tbsp sesame seed oil
- 1/8 tsp ground cinnamon
- ¼ tsp ground cumin
- ½ tsp celery seed
- 1/8 tsp cayenne pepper
- 1 tsp ground coriander
- 2 tbsp sesame seeds

Directions:

1. Preheat the oven to 400° F
2. While the oven is preheating, grease a baking sheet with cooking spray

3. Pull out a frying pan and on low heat fry the sesame seeds while stirring contently

4. After 1 to 2 mins, or the sesame seeds are golden brown, remove the seeds from the heat and set them aside

5. In a large mixing bowl, place the toasted sesame seeds, sesame seed oil, cinnamon, cumin, celery seed, cayenne pepper, and coriander inside and stir until it is mixed evenly

6. Using the prepared baking dish, place the tenderloin on top and evenly space them out

7. Use a brush to lather the tenderloin, on both sides, with the mixture

8. Place the baking sheet inside the oven and let bake for about fifteen mins or until they are no longer pink

9. Take the tenderloin out and serve with a side dish immediately.

Nutrition:

- Calories 248
- Carbs 1g
- Fat 16g
- Protein 26g

Delicious Bacon Delight

Prep Time: 1 hour 35 mins

Servings: 16

Cooking: 1 hour

Ingredients:

- 16 bacon slices
- 2 tbsp erythritol
- 3 oz dark chocolate
- 1 tbsp coconut oil
- ½ tbsp ground cinnamon
- 1 tsp maple extract

Directions:

1. Put the cinnamon with erythritol in a bowl, mix and stir
2. Put the bacon slices on a lined baking sheet and sprinkle cinnamon mix on one side of the slice

3. Flip bacon slices to the other side and sprinkle cinnamon mix over them again
4. Preheat an oven to 275F then introduce the bacon slices and bake for 1 hour
5. Get a pan and heat up with the oil to over medium heat
6. Add chocolate to the oil and stir until it melts
7. Add maple extract; stir, take off the heat and set aside to cool for a short time
8. Take bacon strips out of the oven and set aside to cool down, immerse each bacon strips in the chocolate mix and place them on a parchment paper and leave them to cool down completely.
9. Serve cold.

Nutrition:

- Calories 150
- Fiber 4g
- Carbs 1g
- Protein 3g
- Fat 4g

Squeaky Beef Stroganoff

Prep Time: 10 mins

Servings: 4

Cooking: 30 mins

Ingredients:

- 2 cups of beef strip
- 3 tbsp of olive oil
- 1 tbsp of almond flour
- 1 chopped up onion
- 2 minced up garlic cloves
- 1 cup of sliced mushroom
- 2 tbsp of tomato paste
- 3 tbsp of Worcestershire sauce
- 2 cups of beef broth
- 1 and a ½ cup of zucchini zoodles
- ¼ tsp of flavored vinegar
- ¼ tsp of pepper

Directions:

1. Take a taking a bowl and add in the flavored vinegar, pepper and flour alongside the beef strips
2. Coat up the beef with the flour and the seasoning
3. Set your instant pot on low heat and low pressure and place your meat in your inner pot and cook for 10 mins
4. Add in the rest of your ingredients: in your pot Close up the lid and let it cook for about 18 mins at medium pressure.
5. Once done, release the pressure naturally
6. Serve finally alongside a good bunch of zoodles

Nutrition:

- Calories 335
- Fat: 18g
- Carbs 22g
- Protein 20.02g

Sloppiest Sloppy Joe

Prep Time: 10 mins

Servings: 4

Cooking: 15 mins

Ingredients:

- ½ a cup of white quinoa
- 2 tbsp of olive oil
- 1 large sized chopped up yellow onion
- 1 large sized Italian frying pepper completely stemmed, chopped up and deseeded
- 2 lb of lean ground beef
- 2 tsp of minced up garlic
- 1 pieces of 18 oz can of crushed tomatoes
- ½ cup of old fashioned oat tolls
- ¼ cup of packed dark brown sugar
- 2 tbsp of Dijon mustard
- 2 tbsp of Worcestershire sauce
- 2 tbsp of apple vinegar

- 2 tbsp of paprika
- ¼ tsp of ground clove

Directions:

1. Open up your instant pot and add in the grains
2. Pour in as much water, as required to cover up the grains
3. Lock up the lid and let it cook at high pressure for 3 mins
4. Quick release the pressure
5. Open up and drain out the quinoa in a fine mesh sieve set in your sink
6. Heat up your cooker in sauté mode and pour some oil
7. Add in the pepper, onion and cook for 4 mins
8. Then, add in the crumbled ground beef and garlic and keep stirring them nicely
9. Let it cook for 6 mins until the beef is not pink anymore
10. Then, stir in the tomatoes, brown sugar, oats , mustard, vinegar, cloves, paprika and Worcestershire sauce alongside the nicely drained quinoa to and stir them to mix nicely
11. Close up the lid and let it cook for 8 mins at HIGH pressure

12. Quick release the pressure

13. Open it up and serve hot

Nutrition:

- Calories: 212
- Fat: 14g
- Carbs: 11g
- Protein: 12g

Wrapped Asparagus

Prep Time: 3 mins

Servings: 4

Cooking: 5 mins

Ingredients:

- 1 lb of thick asparagus
- 80 ounce of thinly sliced prosciutto

Directions:

1. The first step here is to prepare your instant pot by pouring in about 2 cups of water
2. Take the asparagus and wrap them up in prosciutto spears.
3. Once all of the asparagus are wrapped, gently place the processed asparaguses in the cooking basket inside your pot in layers.
4. Turn up the heat to a high temperature and when there is a pressure build up, take down the heat and let it cook for about 2-3 mins at the high pressure.

5. Once the timer runs out, gently open the cover of the pressure cooker
6. Take out the steamer basket from the pot instantly and toss the asparaguses on a plate to serve
7. Eat warm or let them come down to room temperature

Nutrition:

- Calories: 212
- Fat: 14g
- Carbohydrates: 11g
- Protein: 12g

Majestic Veal Stew

Prep Time: 10 mins

Servings: 4

Cooking: 30 mins

Ingredients:

- 2 sprigs of fresh rosemary
- 1 tbsp of olive oil
- 1 tbsp of butter
- 8 ounce of shallot
- 2 chopped up carrot
- 2 chopped up stalks of celery
- 2 tbsp of all-purpose flour
- 3 lb of veal
- Water
- 2 tsp of flavored vinegar

Directions:

1. Set your pot to Saute mode and add olive oil, allow the oil to heat up

2. Add butter and chopped up rosemary
3. Add celery, shallots, carrots and Saute until you have a nice texture
4. Shove the veggies on the side and add meat cubes, brown them. Pour stock and cover the meat slightly. Lock up the lid and cook on HIGH pressure for 15-20 mins
5. Release the pressure naturally over 10 mins
6. Open the lid and set the pot to Saute mode, simmer for 5 mins more.

Nutrition:

- Calories 470
- Fat 22g
- Carbs 18g
- Protein 47g

The Surprising No "Noodle" Lasagna

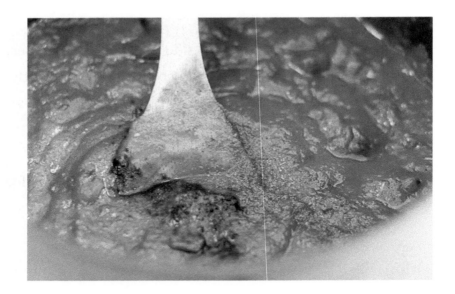

Prep Time: 10 mins

Servings: 8

Cooking: 25 mins

Ingredients:

- 1 lb of ground beef
- 2 cloves of minced garlic
- 1 small sized onion

- 1 and a ½ cups of ricotta cheese
- ½ a cup of parmesan cheese
- 1 large sized egg
- 25 ounce of marinara sauce
- 8 ounce of sliced mozzarella

Directions:

1. Set your pot to Saute mode and add garlic, onion and ground beef
2. Take a small bowl and add ricotta and parmesan with egg and mix
3. Drain the grease and transfer the beef to a 1 and a ½ quart soufflé dish
4. Add marinara sauce to the browned meat and reserve half
5. Top the remaining meat sauce with half of your mozzarella cheese
6. Spread half of the ricotta cheese over the mozzarella layer
7. Top with the remaining meat sauce
8. Add a final layer of mozzarella cheese on top
9. Spread any remaining ricotta cheese mix over the mozzarella
10. Carefully add this mixture to your Soufflé Dish (with meat)

11. Pour 1 cup of water to your pot

12. Place it over a trivet

13. Lock up the lid and cook on HIGH pressure for 10 mins

14. Release the pressure naturally over 10 mins

Nutrition:

- Calories: 607
- Fat: 23g
- Carbohydrates: 65g
- Protein: 33g

Worthwhile Balsamic Beef

Prep Time: 5 mins

Servings: 8

Cooking: 55 mins

Ingredients:

- 3 lb of chuck roast
- 3 cloves of thinly sliced garlic
- 1 tbsp of oil
- 1 tsp of flavored vinegar
- ½ a tsp of pepper
- ½ a tsp of rosemary
- 1 tbsp of butter
- ½ a tsp of thyme
- ¼ cup of balsamic vinegar
- 1 cup of beef broth

Directions:

1. Cut slits in the roast and stuff garlic slices all over

2. Take a bowl and add flavored vinegar, rosemary, pepper, thyme and rub the mixture over the roast. Set your pot to Saute mode and add oil, allow the oil to heat up

3. Add roast and brown both sides (5 mins each side)

4. Take the roast out and keep it on the side

5. Add butter, broth, balsamic vinegar and deglaze the pot

6. Transfer the roast back and lock up the lid, cook on HIGH pressure for 40 mins

7. Preform a quick release

Nutrition:

- Calories: 393
- Fat: 15g
- Carbs: 25g
- Protein: 37g

Lightning Source UK Ltd.
Milton Keynes UK
UKHW020632140621
385477UK00005B/193